LONG-TERM CARE IN MAINE:
HOME AND COMMUNITY-BASED SERVICES

LONG-TERM CARE IN MAINE:
HOME AND COMMUNITY-BASED SERVICES

John V. Lambert
Editor

Novinka Books
New York

Editorial Production Manager: Donna Dennis
Senior Production Editor: Susan Boriotti
Production Editors: Marius Andronie, Rusudan Razmadze and Keti Datunashvili
Office Manager: Annette Hellinger
Graphics: Magdalena Nuñez
Editorial Production: Maya Columbus, Vladimir Klestov, and Lorna Loperfido
Circulation: Ave Maria Gonzalez, Vera Popovic, Luis Aviles, Alexandra Columbus, Raymond Davis, Cathy DeGregory, Melissa Diaz, Marlene Nuñez and Jeannie Pappas

Library of Congress Cataloging-in-Publication Data
Available Upon Request

ISBN: 1-59454-015-2

Nova Science Publishers, Inc.
400 Oser Ave, Suite 1600
Hauppauge, New York 11788-3619
Tele.: 631-231-7269 Fax: 631-231-8175
e-mail: Novascience@earthlink.net
Web Site: http://www.novapublishers.com

Printed in the United States of America

CONTENTS

PREFACE

Demographic challenges posed by the growing elderly population and demands for greater public commitment to home and community-based care for persons with disabilities have drawn the attention of federal and state policymakers for some time. Spending on long-term care by both the public and private sectors is significant. In 2001, spending for long-term care services for persons of all ages represented 12.2% of all personal health care spending (almost $152 billion of $1.24 trillion). Federal and state governments accounted for almost two-thirds of all spending. By far, the primary payer for long-term care is the federal-state Medicaid program, which paid for almost half of all U.S. long-term care spending in 2001.

Federal and state Medicaid spending for long-term care in FY2001 was about $75 billion, representing over one-third of all Medicaid spending. Over 70% of Medicaid long-term care spending was for institutions — nursing homes and intermediate care facilities for the mentally retarded (ICFs/MR). Many believe that the current federal financing system paid through Medicaid is structurally biased in favor of institutional care. State governments face significant challenges in refocusing care systems, given the structure of current federal financing. Many states have devoted significant efforts to change their long-term care systems to expand home and community-based services for persons with disabilities and their families. Nevertheless, financing of nursing home care — primarily through the Medicaid program — still dominates most states' spending on long-term care today.

While some advocates maintain that the federal government should play a larger role in providing support for home and community-based care, Congress has not yet decided whether or how to change current federal policy. One possibility is that Congress may continue an incremental approach to long-term care, without major federal policy involvement, leaving to state governments the responsibility for developing strategies that support home and community-based care within existing federal funding constraints and program rules.

To help Congress review various policy alternatives and to assist policymakers understand issues that states face in development of long-term care services, the Congressional Research Service (CRS) undertook a study of ten states in 2002. The research was undertaken to look at state policies on long-term care as well as trends in both institutional and home and community-based care for persons with disabilities (the elderly, persons with mental retardation, and other adults with disabilities). The research included a review of state documents and data on long-term care, as well as national data sources on spending. Interviews were held with state officials responsible for long-term care, a wide range of stakeholders and, in some cases, members or staff of state legislatures.

The 10 states included in the study are: Arizona, Florida, Illinois, Indiana, Louisiana, Maine, Oklahoma, Oregon, Pennsylvania, and Texas. States were chosen according to a number of variables, including geographic distribution, demographic trends, and approaches to financing, administration and delivery of long-term care services.

This section presents background and analysis about long-term care in Maine.

Chapter 1

INTRODUCTION: FEDERAL LEGISLATIVE PERSPECTIVE*

The Social Security Amendments of 1965, which created the Medicaid program, required states to provide skilled nursing facility services, under their state Medicaid plans, and gave nursing home care the same level of priority as hospital and physician services:

> "Section 1902 (a) A State plan for medical assistance must provide for inclusion of some institutional and some noninstitutional care and services, and, effective July 1, 1967, provide (A) for inclusion of at least (1) inpatient hospital services… ; (2) outpatient hospital services, (3) other laboratory and X-ray services; (4) skilled nursing home services (other than services in an institution for tuberculosis or mental diseases) for individuals 21 years of age or older, (5) physicians services… ;" P.L. 89-97, July 30, 1965.

States choosing to modify their programs for long-term care face significant challenges. Financing of nursing home care has dominated long-term care spending for decades. The federal financing structure that created incentives to support institutional care reaches back to 1965. A number of converging factors have supported reliance on nursing home spending. Prior to enactment of Medicaid, homes for the aged and other public institutions were financed by a combination of direct payments made by individuals with their Social Security Old Age Assistance (OAA) benefits, and vendor

---

* Excerpted from CRS Report RL32166 by Jane Tilly, Carol O'Shaughnessy and Rob Weissert

payments made by states with federal matching payments on behalf of individuals. The Kerr-Mills Medical Assistance to the Aged (MAA) program, enacted in 1960, a predecessor to Medicaid, allowed states to provide medical services, including skilled nursing home services, to persons who were not eligible for OAA cash payments, thereby expanding the eligible population.[1]

In 1965, when Kerr-Mills was transformed into the federal-state Medicaid program, Congress created an *entitlement* to skilled nursing facility care under the expanded program. The Social Security Amendments of 1965 required that states provide skilled nursing facility services and gave nursing home care the same level of priority as hospital and physician services. Amendments in 1967 allowed states to provide care in "intermediate care facilities" (ICFs) for persons who did not need skilled nursing home care, but needed more than room and board. In 1987, Congress eliminated the distinction between skilled nursing facilities and intermediate care facilities (effective in 1990). As a result of these various amendments, people eligible under the state's Medicaid plan are *entitled* to nursing home facility care; that is, if a person meets the state's income and asset requirements, as well as the state's functional eligibility requirements for entry into a nursing home, he or she is entitled to the benefit.

Since its inception, Medicaid has been the predominant payor for nursing home care. In 1970, over $1 billion was spent on nursing home care through Medicaid and Medicare. Federal and state Medicaid payments accounted for almost all of this spending. 87% Medicaid spending for nursing home care grew by 50% in the three year period beginning in 1967.

In FY2001, Medicaid spent $53.1 billion on institutional care for nursing homes and care in intermediate care facilities for the mentally retarded).

These early legislative developments were the basis for the beginnings of the modern day nursing home industry. Significant growth in the number of nursing homes occurred during the 1960s — from 1960 to 1970, the number of homes more than doubled, from 9,582 to almost 23,000, and the

---

[1] CRS Report 83-181, *Nursing Home Legislation: Issues and Policies,* by Maureen Baltay. Archived and available upon request from the Congressional Research Service (CRS).

number of beds more than tripled, from 331,000 to more than one million.[2] (Today there are about 17,000 nursing homes with 1.8 million beds.[3])

During the latter part of the 1960s and the 1970s, nursing home care attracted a great deal of congressional oversight as a result of concern about increasing federal expenditures, and a pattern of instances of fraud and abuse that was becoming evident. Between 1969 and 1976, the Subcommittee on Long-Term Care of the Senate special committee on Aging, held 30 hearings on problems in the nursing home industry.[4]

Home care services received some congressional attention in the authorizing statute — home health care services were one of the optional services that states could provide under the 1965 law. Three years later in 1968, Congress amended the law to require states to provide home health care services to persons entitled to skilled nursing facility care as part of their state Medicaid plans (effective in 1970). During the 1970s, the Department of Health, Education and Welfare (now Health and Human Services, DHHS) devoted attention to "alternatives to nursing home care" through a variety of federal research and demonstration efforts. These efforts were undertaken not only to find ways to offset the high costs of nursing facility care, but also to respond to the desires of persons with disabilities to remain in their homes and in community settings, rather than in institutions. However, it was not until 1981 that Congress took significant legislative action to expand home and community-based services through Medicaid when it authorized the Medicaid Section 1915(c) home and community-based waiver program.

Under that authority (known then as the Section 2176 waiver program), the Secretary of DHHS may waive certain Medicaid state plan requirements to allow states to cover a wide range of home and community-based services to persons who otherwise meet the state's eligibility requirements for institutional care. The waiver provision was designed to alter the fact that the Medicaid program had emphasized institutional care rather than care in home and community-based settings. Services under the Section 1915(c)

---

2 U.S. Congress, Senate Special Committee on Aging, Developments in Aging, 1970, Report 92-46, Feb. 16, 1970, Washington, cited from the *American Nursing Home Association Fact Book, 1969-1970.*

3 American Health Care Association, *Facts and Trends 2001, The Nursing Facility Sourcebook*, 2001, Washington. The number of nursing homes is for 1999 2000 and number of beds is for 1998. (Hereafter cited as American Health Care Association, *The Nursing Facility Sourcebook.*)

4 U.S. Congress, Senate Special Committee on Aging, *Nursing Home Care in the United States: Failure of Public Policy,* Washington, 1974, and supporting papers published in succeeding years.

waiver include: case management, personal care, homemaker, home health aide, adult day care, habilitation, environmental modifications, among many others.[5] These services are covered as an *option* of states, and under the law, persons are not entitled to these services as they are to nursing facility care. Moreover, states are allowed to set cost caps and limits on the numbers and types of persons to be served under their waiver programs.

Notwithstanding wide use of the Section 1915(c) waiver authority by states over the last two decades, total spending for Medicaid home and community-based services waivers is significantly less than institutional care — about $14.4 billion in 2001, compared to $53.1 billion for nursing facility care services and care for persons with mental retardation in intermediate care facilities (ICFs/MR). Despite this disparity in spending, in many states the Section 1915(c) waiver program is the primary source of financial support for a wide range of home and community-based services, and funding has been increasing steadily. Federal and state Medicaid support for the waiver programs increased by over 807% from FY1990 to FY2001 (in constant 2001 dollars).

The home and community-based waiver program has been a significant source of support to care for persons with mental retardation and developmental disabilities as states have closed large state institutions for these persons over the last two decades. Nationally, in FY2001, almost 75% of Section 1915(c) waiver funding was devoted to providing services to these individuals.

---

[5] States may waive the following Medicaid requirements: (1) statewideness — states may cover services in only a portion of the state, rather than in all geographic jurisdictions; (2) comparability of services — states may cover state-selected groups of persons, rather than all persons otherwise eligible. In addition, states may use more liberal income requirements for persons needing home and community-based waiver services than would otherwise apply to persons living in the community. For further information, see CRS Report RL31163, *Long-Term Care: A Profile of Medicaid 1915(c) Home and Community-based Services Waivers,* by Carol O'Shaughnessy and Rachel Kelly.

States administer their long-term care programs against this backdrop of federal legislative initiatives — first, the *entitlement* to nursing home care, and requirement to provide home health services to persons entitled to nursing home care, and, second, the *option* to provide a wide range of home and community-based services through waiver of federal law, within state-defined eligibility requirements, service availability, and limits on numbers of persons served.

Chapter 2

SUMMARY OVERVIEW[1]

OVERVIEW

Maine has pursued an aggressive policy to decrease dependence on nursing homes as a result of a 1993 budgetary crisis involving rapidly escalating Medicaid nursing home costs. Its policies to tighten nursing home eligibility and expand community options have decreased reliance on nursing homes dramatically.

Maine has also decreased its reliance on institutions for persons with developmental disabilities. The state closed its large state-operated facility in 1995, and has greatly reduced its use of private intermediate care facilities for the mentally retarded (ICFs/MR). Care of this population has shifted to the home and smaller group residential settings.

DEMOGRAPHIC TRENDS

Maine is one of the smallest states in the country with 1.27 million people in 2000; its population increased by 50,000 people during the 1990s. It also is one of the oldest states, with 14.4% of its population aged 65 and older. In 2025, 21.4% of Maine's population will be age 65 years or older, compared to 18.5% for the nation.

---

[1] Information based on Maine data and documents, national data, and interviews with state officials. This section does not discuss programs for persons with mental illness. It also generally excludes discussion of programs for infants and children with disabilities, other than those serving persons with mental retardation and developmental disabilities.

Persons aged 85 and over with two or more limitations in activities of daily living are estimated to increase 15.3% by 2010 to reach 2,047; the number of persons aged 18 to 64 with the same level of disability will increase by 6% reaching 2,990.

Administration of Long-Term Care Programs

Responsibility for administration and management of long-term care services for persons with disabilities is spread across several state agencies, with the Department of Human Services (DHS) retaining responsibility for most programs. Various sub-state agencies and some private contractors have responsibility for different aspects of long-term care administration and services.

Maine uses several management tools to try to control use of nursing homes and to manage its home and community-based services including: 1) pre-admission screening for all nursing home applicants, 2) contracted assessment and case management agencies for adults receiving home care agency services, and 3) a separate agency for participants in consumer-directed, personal assistance programs.

Trends in Institutional Care

Between 1995 and 2001, according to state data, the percentage of public long-term care beneficiaries served in nursing homes declined from 50% to 33%. During the same time period, the percentage of public long-term care funding devoted to these facilities decreased from 84% to 61%.

Very few persons with mental retardation and developmental disabilities who live in residential settings live in large institutions; in 2002, 10% of persons in residential settings lived in settings serving seven or more persons. Persons living in small residential settings (with six or fewer persons) has increased from 62% of all persons living in group residential settings in 1991 to over 90% in 2002. This is due in part to expanded use of Maine’s Section 1915(c) home and community-based waiver program which was designed to move people from large institutions into smaller settings.

TRENDS IN HOME AND COMMUNITY-BASED CARE

In FY2001, Maine provided about 5,000 older persons and persons with disabilities with the following Medicaid state plan services: private duty nursing, home health, personal care, and adult day care. In addition, the state relies on two Medicaid Section 1915(c) home and community based waivers to serve the adult population with disabilities — the Elder and Adult Waiver and the Consumer-Directed Waiver. Together they served about 2,000 participants in FY2001. The state also has a large Medicaid and state-funded residential care program which served about 4,300 persons in FY2001. The largest state funded program is Home-Based Care, which served about 4,000 people in FY2001.

Maine uses one optional Medicaid state plan service — day habitation; one Medicaid Section 1915(c) home and community-based services waiver, which includes day habitation; and some state-funded programs to serve persons with developmental disabilities. The state's Section 1915(c) waiver serves people who would otherwise be in an institution. It provides residential training in licensed homes, personal support, day habilitation, supported employment, respite, environmental modification, crisis intervention, and other services. About 2,200 people received services in FY2002.

LONG-TERM CARE SPENDING

Long-term care comprises a significant portion of Medicaid spending in Maine — about 30% of all Medicaid spending was devoted to long-term care in FY2001 ($411 million out of $1.3 billion). Nursing home spending represented 15% of all Medicaid spending.

As a share of Medicaid long term care spending, nursing home spending decreased from 65.5% to 49% from FY1990-FY2001. During the same time period, Medicaid spending for institutions for persons with mental retardation decreased from 23.2% to 10.9%.

In FY2001, Maine spent $152.8 million on Medicaid Section 1915(c) home and community-based services waiver programs, a 536% increase (in constant 2001 dollars) from FY1990.

ISSUES IN FINANCING AND DELIVERY OF LONG-TERM CARE

One of the challenges Maine faces during its 2003 budgetary crisis is to hold on to the gains it has made in providing home and community services to people with disabilities, while dealing with its fiscal constraints.

The labor shortage is a critical problem affecting all areas of health care, including long-term care for older persons and care for persons with developmental disabilities, particularly in Southern Maine. The labor shortage also makes it difficult to recruit state and privately-employed case managers.

Much of the state is rural and it is a challenge for people to travel to services or for workers to get to the homes of people with disabilities. Transportation services is a largely unmet need in these areas.

Chapter 3

DEMOGRAPHIC TRENDS

Maine is one of the smallest states in the country with 1.27 million people in 2000; the population increased by about 50,000 people in the past decade. It also is one of the oldest states, with 14.4% of its population aged 65 and older — more than 183,000 people in 2000. The state's older population is growing quite rapidly; it rose 12.3% during the 1990s. Those most in need of long-term care — the population age 85 and older — grew by 27.9% during the same time period (**Table 1**). Almost one-third of non-institutionalized persons age 65 and older live alone.

Table 1. Maine Population Age 65 and Older, 1990 and 2000

Age	1990		2000		1990-2000 percent change	2000 population rank in U.S. (based on %)
	Number	% of total population	Number	% of population		
65+	163,373	13,3	183,402	14.4%	12.3%	7
65-74	91,600	7.5	96,196	7.5%	5.0%	4
75-84	53,547	4.4	63,890	5.0%	19.3%	9
85+	18,226	1.5	23,316	1.8%	27.9%	45
Under 65	1,064,555	86.7	1,091,521	85.6%	2.5%	45
Total	**1,227,928**		**1,274,923**		**3.85**	**40**

Source: U.S. Census Bureau, *Profile of General Demographics for Maine: 1990. 2000* at [http://www.census.gov/census2000/state/me.html]. Numbers may not sum to 100 due to rounding.

Maine, along with the rest of the country, will experience large increases in its older population over the next 25 years. By 2025, its elderly population will have increased by 77.3% (see **Figure 1**). In 2025, 21.4% of Maine's population will be aged 65 years or older, compared to 18.5% for the nation

(**Table 2**). Maine will have to address the long-term care needs of 300,000 elderly in that year, 30,000 of whom will be aged 85 or older.

Table 2. Elderly Population as a Percent of Total Population, Maine and the United States, 2025

Age	Percent of total population, Maine	Percent of total population, United States
65+	21.4%	18.5%
65-74	12.8%	10.5%
75-84	6.6%	5.8%
85+	2.0%	2.2%
Under 65 population	78.6%	81.5%

Source: CRS calculations based on data from the U.S. Census Bureau. Projections at [http://www.gov/population/www/projections/st_urby5.html]; analyzed data from State Populations Projections: Every Fifth Year. See **Appendix 3** for information about projection assumptions.

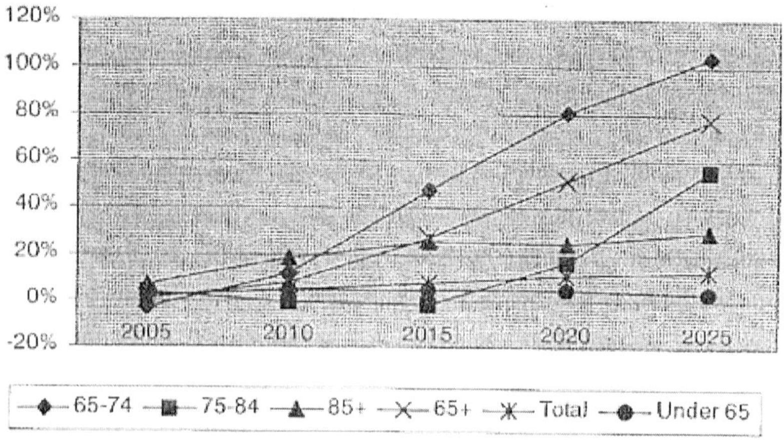

Figure 1. Projected Percentage Population Increases in Maine Over 2000 by Population for Selected Years, 2000-2025.

Source: CRS calculations based on data from the U.S. Census Bureau, Projections at [http://www.census.gov/populations/st_yrby5.html]; analyzed data from State Populations Projections: Every Fifth Year.

NEED FOR LONG-TERM CARE

Table 3 presents estimates of the number of persons aged 18 and over in Maine who have limitations in two or more activities of daily living (ADLs) and thus may need long-term care. These estimates were derived from data generated by The Lewin Group and combine national level data on persons with disabilities with state-level data from the U.S. Census Bureau on age, income, and broad measures of disability. Persons aged 85 and over with two or more limitations in ADLs are estimated to increase 15.3% by 2010 to reach 2,047. The number of persons aged 18 to 64 with the same level of disability will increase by 6% reaching almost 3,000. Growth in the number of adults of all ages with disabilities will place pressure on public and private long-term care resources.

Table 3. Estimated Number of Persons with Two or More Limitations in Activities of Daily Living (ADLs), by Poverty Status, in Maine

Percent of poverty	Persons with 2+ADI limitations by age and income								
	2002			2005			2010		
	18-64	65+	85+	18-64	65+	85+	18-64	65+	85+
Up to 100%	597	742	128	613	752	134	634	796	148
Up to 150%	954	1,984	738	979	2,027	771	1,014	2,159	852
Up to 200%	1,234	2,770	1,070	1,276	2,830	1,119	1,321	3,032	1,235
All income	2,822	5,239	1,775	2,894	5,343	1,854	2,990	5,707	2,047

Source: CRS analysis based on projections generated by The Lewin Group through the HCBS State-by-State Population Tool available on-line at [http://www.lewin.com/cltc]. Lisa M.B. Alecxih, and Ryan Foreman, *The Lewin Group Center on Long Term Care HCBS Population Tool*, 2002.

Chapter 4

ADMINISTRATION OF LONG-TERM CARE PROGRAMS

Responsibility for administration and management of long-term care services for persons with disabilities is spread across several state agencies, with the Department of Human Services (DHS) retaining responsibility for most programs. Various sub-state agencies and some private contractors have responsibility for different aspects of long-term care administration and services.

The *Department of Human Services* is the single state agency for Medicaid; and three of its bureaus administer most of the state's long-term care programs. The Bureau of Medical Services (BMS) is the fiscal agent for Medicaid; it processes claims, enrolls participating providers, and manages Medicaid's optional personal care service. The Bureau of Elder and Adult Services (BEAS) manages two of the state's four Medicaid Section 1915(c) home and community-based services waivers along with Medicaid home health and private duty nursing, nursing home eligibility determination and some of the residential options. The Bureau of Family Independence (BFT) determines financial eligibility for all Medicaid applicants.

The *Department of Behavioral and Developmental Services (DBDS)* houses the Bureau of Adult Mental Retardation Services, which manages one waiver, day habilitation, and a number of state-funded services for persons with developmental disabilities. The waiver is managed in partnership with the DHS.

The *Department of Labor (DoL)* gained responsibility for administering the state's consumer-directed programs in 2002, including the Medicaid personal care optional service for those who want to direct their own services, the consumer-directed Medicaid Section 1915(c) home and community-based services waiver, and the state-funded consumer-directed program.

The DHS Division of Licensing and Certification licenses nursing homes and ICFs/MR. Until 2001, the Division also licensed assisted living facilities (ALFs). This responsibility went to BEAS because the state wanted to maintain the social model for ALFs in contrast to the medical model that the Department used when it regulated those facilities.

RESPONSIBILITY FOR ASSESSMENT, ELIGIBILITY, AND CASE MANAGEMENT

Maine uses several management tools to try to control use of nursing homes and to manage its home and community-based services including: 1) pre-admission screening for nursing home applicants using a standardized assessment tool, 2) contracted assessment and case management agencies for adults receiving agency-provided home care services, and 3) a contracted agency that assists participants in consumer-directed programs.

Functional Eligibility

A private agency — Goold Data Management — conducts the assessments of functional eligibility and authorizes service plans that establish the amount and type of services for all persons receiving Medicaid home and community-based services. After this assessment, people are advised of what their long-term care options are and many are able to remain in the community or enter group residential settings rather than enter a nursing home. Fifty-four nurses statewide conducted 16,359 assessments in State Fiscal Year (SFY) 2001 at a cost of $153 per assessment.[1] State officials and stakeholders commented that people who receive Medicaid home health services from certified home health agencies must have two assessments, the state's uniform assessment as well as the Outcome and Assessment Information Set (OASIS) tool that is federally required when people receive Medicare or Medicaid-funded home health services. Some stakeholders advocate replacing the state's tool with OASIS, but state

[1] Bureau of Elder and Adult Services, Maine's Home and Community-Based Care System, at [www.state.me.as.dhs/ltc/2000], accessed on Feb. 6, 2002.

officials resist this idea because they believe their tool meets their management needs better than OASIS would.

Financial Eligibility

The Bureau of Family Independence handles the financial eligibility determination for Medicaid services through its 15 local offices. Some interviewees said that financial eligibility standards for long-term care programs differ and are so complex that applicants cannot understand them; BEAS staff say they help people work through the eligibility rules so that they obtain the benefits for which they qualify. However, some stakeholders complained that the determination process can take several months, which delays receipt of services. State officials say that financial eligibility determination generally takes place within 45 days of submission of the forms; complex financial situations can take longer to process.

Care Coordination and Consumer-Directed Services

In 1996, Elder Independence of Maine (EIM), which is a division of the Western Maine Area Agency on Aging, began providing care coordination services (i.e., arranging and monitoring services) to persons across the state who receive Medicaid and state-funded home and community-based services. EIM receives a monthly per capita payment of $117 to arrange services, coordinate and monitor care, calculate consumer copayments, contract with service providers, pay claims, audit providers, and participate in quality improvement activities. EIM contracted with 200 providers and served 6,825 consumers in SFY2001 in four programs.

Maine has established a consumer-directed program where persons with disabilities plan their care, including services and providers of their choice. The state contracts out management of its consumer-directed programs to Alpha One, Maine's Center for Independent Living (CIL). Alpha One conducts assessments for people seeking to direct their own services and coordinates the state's three consumer-directed programs. The CIL provides consumer skills training, monitoring, and payroll processing for consumers. In SFY2001, Alpha One served 357 consumers eligible under the state's Medicaid consumer-directed program and received payments of $132 per consumer per month; it also served 297 consumers eligible under the state's

Section 1915(c) waiver program and received payments of $335 per consumer per month.[2]

The Department of Behavioral and Developmental Services performs case management for its clients with developmental disabilities through its three regional offices. Case managers are state employees who, in addition to assessing eligibility and developing service plans, also visit people in nursing homes to determine if they can live in the community in small group homes, for example. About 4,500 people receive case management services from the Department. After a person is determined eligible and has a service plan, the provider agency takes over most day-to-day case management functions, in addition to providing services.

2 Personal communication with staff of the Maine Department of Labor, June 6, 2003.

Chapter 5

MAINE'S LONG-TERM CARE SERVICES FOR THE ELDERLY AND PERSONS WITH DISABILITIES

TRENDS IN INSTITUTIONAL CARE

Maine has pursued an aggressive policy to decrease dependence on nursing homes in its long-term care system. The state started on this course because of a 1993 budgetary crisis. Since nursing home costs had increased by 50% over a 3-year period,[1] the state implemented stringent functional eligibility criteria for Medicaid nursing home care in 1994. Prior to implementation of these criteria, people had been able to obtain Medicaid nursing home coverage if they needed assistance with one activity of daily living (ADL) or one instrumental activity of daily living (IADL).[2] According to some stakeholders, the new criteria resulted in some people being released to or remaining in the community without sufficient home and community service alternatives. According to interviewees, the Alzheimer's Association succeeded in amending the functional criteria for nursing home eligibility to

---

1 Bureau of Elder and Adult Services, *Long-Term Care Reform in Maine.*

2 The need for long-term care assistance is measured by assessing a person's need for assistance with *activities of daily living (ADLs)* and/or *instrumental activities of daily living (IADLs).* ADLs are activities necessary to carry out basic human functions, and include the following: bathing, dressing, eating, getting around inside the home, toileting, and transferring from a bed to a chair. *IADLs* are tasks necessary for independent community living, and include the following: shopping, light housework, laundry, taking medication, telephoning, money management, and meal preparation.

define nursing need to include management of cognition and behavior. The standard now requires an applicant to need a form of therapy 5 days a week, assistance with three specific ADLs, nursing services three times a week, or have a cognitive or behavior problem.

In 1994, the Maine legislature adopted a policy of universal pre-admission screening of all nursing home applicants so facilities cannot admit anyone unless they first have an assessment. The state found that there were not enough residential alternatives to nursing homes, and that waiting lists for home and community services had developed. To ameliorate this situation, in 1996, the state devoted more funding to home and community services. As a result, Medicaid nursing home admissions decreased and use of home and community services increased. (**Tables 4** and **5**). Between 1995 and 2001, the percentage of publicly-funded, aged and disabled long-term care beneficiaries served in nursing homes declined from 50% to 33%. During the same time period the percentage of public long-term care funding devoted to these facilities decreased from 84% to 61%.

Table 4. Where People Receive Publicly Funded Long-Term Care Services

	1995	2001
Total served in all settings	19,803	25,455
Home care	39%	49%
Assisted living	11%	18%
Nursing homes	50%	33%

Source: Calculations based on the Bureau of Elder and Adult Services, Dec. 27, 2001, as revised on Feb. 7, 2002.

Table 5. Where Public Long-Term Care Funding Goes

	1995	2001
Funds spent in all settings	$284,715,157	$328,581,664
Home care	10%	20%
Assisted living	6%	19%
Nursing homes	84%	61%

Source: Calculations based on the Bureau of Elder and Adult Services, Dec. 27, 2001, as revised on Feb. 7, 2002.

In 2000, Maine had 126 nursing facilities with 8,236 beds, with an occupancy rate of 88.7% (**Table 6**). The number of beds per 1,000 older persons (44.9) is lower than the national average (52.7). The state's ratio for persons aged 85 and older is 353.2 beds per 1,000, a figure much lower than the national rate of 434.8. The relatively high occupancy rates combined with the low ratio of nursing home beds to older persons, implies that the state does not have much excess capacity in its nursing home industry. According to data supplied by officials from the Maine Bureau of Medical Services, Medicaid helps fund the costs of 72% of all nursing home residents.

Table 6. Nursing Home Characteristics in Maine and the United States

Characteristics	Maine	United States
Number of facilities	126	17,023
Number of residents	7,309	1,490,155
Number of beds	8,236	1,843,522
Number of Medicaid beds	6,497	841,458
Number of beds per 1,000 pop. aged 65 and older	44.9	52.7
Number of beds per 1,000 pop. aged 75 and older	94.4	111.1
Number of beds per 1,000 pop. aged 85 and older	353.2	434.8
Occupancy rate	88.7%	80.8%

Source: CRS calculations based on data from the American Health Care Association (ACHA), *Facts and Trends: The Nursing Facility Sourcebook*, 2001. All figures represent 1999-2000 data.

Some stakeholders claim that about half of nursing facilities are technically insolvent due to low payment rates and a handful have closed in recent years. State officials counter that Maine has one of the highest nursing home payment rates in the country. Officials mentioned that elimination of the Boren amendment, which required that state Medicaid nursing home payment rates be "reasonable and adequate to meet the costs which must be incurred by efficiently and economically operated facilities" (Section 1902(a)(13) of the Social Security Act), enabled the state to control payments to nursing homes and avoid paying unnecessary costs.

Nursing home quality is said to be generally good. According to interviewees, since many homes are located in rural areas where people know one another well, the resulting sense of community promotes delivery of good quality care. In some rural communities, the facilities are a major employer in the area.

TRENDS IN HOME AND COMMUNITY-BASED CARE

Maine takes advantage of Medicaid's mandatory and optional state plan services as well as Section 1915(c) waivers to provide home and community-based care to adults with disabilities. In FY2001, the state provided about 5,000 participants with the following Medicaid state plan services: private duty nursing, home health, personal care, and adult day care. Costs of these services in FY2001 were $19.4 million. In addition, the state relies on two waivers to serve the adult population with disabilities in home and community-based settings — the Elder and Adult Waiver and the Consumer-directed waiver. Together they served almost 2,000 participants at a cost of $27 million in FY2001. The state also has a large residential care program funded by Medicaid and state funds, which served about 4,300 persons in FY2001.

The state also sponsors a number of programs that do not receive federal funding, most of which serve just a few hundred people. By far the largest program is Home-Based Care, which served about 4,000 people at a cost of $15 million in FY2001. This program and the state's other home and community-based programs for adults have separate consumer-directed components that mirror the main programs.

MEDICAID STATE PLAN SERVICES AND 1915 (C) WAIVERS

Maine's Medicaid mandatory and optional long-term services have varying functional eligibility standards, but all have the same financial eligibility standards. Under the state's Medicaid program, a person's countable income cannot exceed 100% of the federal poverty level. Countable assets cannot exceed $2,000,[3] although the state can disregard an additional $8,000 in financial assets when calculating financial eligibility.

Section 1915(c) waiver services require that a person meet the state's functional eligibility criteria for nursing facility coverage. The income eligibility standard for these waivers is 222% of the federal poverty level and

---

[3] In addition, Medicaid statute requires that certain items are excluded from assets: an individual's home; up to $2,000 of household goods and personal effects; life insurance policies with a face value of $1,500 or less; an automobile with value up to $14,500; and burial funds up to $1,500, among other things.

countable assets cannot exceed $2,000, or $10,000 including an $8,000 additional asset disregard.

Mandatory and Optional State Plan Services

The mandatory state plan *home health* service requires beneficiaries of any age to have a need for skilled care and to be homebound; physicians must order the service. Available services are nursing, therapies, aides, and psychiatric monitoring. There is no cap on the amount of care available to an individual. About 2,000 adults received these services in FY2001 at a cost of $5.3 million.

Private duty nursing and personal care, both optional services under the Maine state Medicaid plan, require beneficiaries of any age to need assistance in at least two of seven activities of daily living (ADLs) or need direction with four ADLs. Both services offer nursing, home health aide, and personal care assistance. Costs are limited to $3,884 a month in FY2001 for people needing a nursing home level of care, but the cost cap for beneficiaries who are dependent on a ventilator is $20,100 a month. The programs served about 2,500 adults in FY2001; the cost of the two programs was $9.3 million in that year.

Consumer-Directed Personal Care is an optional service for persons age 18 and over who need assistance with two of seven ADLs but who are cognitively capable of directing their own services. The service limit is 35 hours a week of daytime care and 14 hours of night-time care. In FY2001, Alpha One served 357 consumers at a cost of $4.1 million.

Adult day health services, another Medicaid optional service under the clinic option, serves people who are age 18 or older and who attend day care a minimum of four hours a week. Services available to the 173 participants (FY2001) include health care monitoring, nursing, rehabilitation counseling, and health promotion. The functional and financial eligibility standards for this service are the same as for private duty nursing and personal care. Adult day health spending was $787,000 in FY2001.

Medicaid Section 1915(c) Waivers

Maine has two Section 1915(c) waivers for the adult population, one for services provided through home care agencies services and the other for consumer-directed services. (The Section 1915(c) waiver for persons with mental retardation is discussed below.) They are administered independently of one another. The *Elder and Adult with Disabilities Waiver* is for persons aged 18 and older who receive a range of services including case management; nursing, aide, and personal care services; therapies; homemaker; adult day care; mental health; and transportation services. The cap on services is 100% of the average nursing facility payment. Elder Independence of Maine administers these waivers.

The *Consumer-Directed Waiver* also serves people who are eligible for nursing facility care, but who are cognitively capable of directing their services. This waiver provides case management, skills training, and personal care assistance. The cap on services is 90% of the average nursing facility payment. As of June 2003, the state was considering exploring an amendment to its Medicaid waiver that would increase the cost cap. The waiver served 279 participants at a cost of $8.3 million in FY2001. Alpha One manages this waiver.

One of the state's largest Medicaid programs is the *Residential Care Services Program,* which paid for the medical and remedial component of group residential care for 4,325 participants in FY2001 at a cost of $45.1 million. State funds paid for the room and board component for most participants accounting for $17 million in the same year. The state expanded this program as it sought to increase alternatives to nursing home care during its budget crisis in the mid-1990s.

Medicaid finances the care component of services in residential care homes (adult family care homes and residential care homes), which have private or shared rooms and baths; and assisted living facilities, which have private apartments. Medicaid payments for residents of all residential facilities are adjusted for varying categories (15 case-mix groups), using a standardized assessment of all residents. Assisted living facility residents receive an average subsidy of $10,657 per year in SFY2003. According to data supplied by the Bureau of Medical Services, Medicaid helps fund the costs of 67% of ALF residents.

Residents who are eligible for Supplemental Security Income (SSI) use these payments and their SSI state supplemental payments to fund their room and board costs. Those who are not SSI eligible must pay 40% of their income and 3% of liquid assets over $10,000 as a co-payment for residential care.

State Programs

There are a number of pathways that establish Medicaid eligibility for home and community-based long-term care services. These include coverage of persons whose income is 300% of the federal Supplemental Security Income (SSI) payment level, as allowed under the Section 1915(c) waiver program ($1,656 a month for an individual in 2003). Despite the availability of this more liberal standard, many people may need community care but cannot meet Medicaid's income limits or resource tests. Many of these persons cannot establish eligibility until they spend-down almost all of their resources and income to meet that eligibility level, and, by that time, may be in danger of entering an institution. One of the issues many states have confronted is how to serve these people.

Maine has addressed this issue in part through its seven state-funded programs. Many of these programs are designed to complement their Medicaid counterparts with more generous financial eligibility standards than those of Medicaid.

By far the largest program is *Home-based Care* for adults aged 18 and over. Eligibility for services is based on the presence of limitations in ADLs and IADLs with at least one being an ADL or if they need direction with four ADLs. The program has no upper limits on participants' incomes or assets. However, the program has a copayment of 4% of monthly income and 3% of assets exceeding $15,000. The program offers a wide array of services including case management, nursing, home health aide, therapies, personal care, and adult day care. These are the same basic services provided under the Elder and Adult Waiver. There are four levels of care with corresponding maximum caps. The cap on services for the highest level is 85% of the nursing facility rate. Elder Independence of Maine runs the program, which served 3,863 persons in FY2001 at a cost of $12.4 million.

In addition, the program has a separately-managed consumer-directed component with the same basic eligibility standards as the agency-provided service program; the service cap is set at 35 hours per week plus 14 hours per week of night personal care services. The consumer-directed component, managed by Alpha One, served 203 people in FY2001 at a cost of $3.1 million.

The state has five other state funded programs — adult day services, congregate housing, assisted living, Alzheimer's respite, and homemaker services — all of which have similar functional and financial eligibility standards as the other two state-funded programs. These five programs served a total of 2,672 participants at a cost of $6 million in FY2001.

Chapter 6

Maine's Long-Term Care Services for Persons with Mental Retardation and Developmental Disabilities

Overview

Services to persons with mental retardation and other developmental disabilities in the United States changed dramatically over the last half of the 20th century as a result of a number of converging factors. These include the advocacy efforts of families and organized constituency groups, various changes to the Social Security law that provided payments to individuals through Supplemental Security Income (SSI) and Supplemental Security Disability Insurance (SSDI) and to service providers through the Medicaid program, and significant litigation brought on behalf of persons with mental retardation.[1]

---

[1] For a detailed history of the development of services for persons with developmental disabilities, see David Braddock, Richard Hemp, Susan Parish, and James Westrich, *The State of the States in Developmental Disabilities*, University of Illinois at Chicago. American Association on Mental Retardation, Washington, DC, 1998. (Hereafter cited as Braddock, et al., *The State of the States in Developmental Disabilities.*)

TRENDS IN INSTITUTIONAL CARE

The early history of services to persons with mental retardation is characterized by the development of large state institutions or training schools begun during the latter part of the 19th century and continuing through the first part of the 20th century. Between 1920 and 1967, institutions quadrupled in size and peaked at almost 200,000 individuals nationwide in 165 free-standing, state-operated mental retardation institutional facilities.[2] Today, some states are still faced with the legacy of large state-operated institutions.

Maine has eliminated its sole large state-operated facility for persons with mental retardation and developmental disabilities. It is also making strides to downsize its other three smaller state-operated facilities (see **Appendix Table 2** for a list of the facilities).

Very few persons with mental retardation and developmental disabilities who live in residential settings live in large institutions; in 2002, 10% of persons in residential settings lived in settings serving 7 or more persons. Persons living in small residential settings (with six or fewer persons) has increased from 62% of all persons living in group residential settings in 1991 to over 90% in 2002 (**Table 7**). This is due in part to expanded use of Maine's Section 1915(c) home and community-based waiver program which was designed to move people from large institutions into smaller settings.

Table 7. Persons with Mental Retardation and Developmental Disabilities Served in Residential Settings, by Size of Setting, 1991, 1995 and 2002

	Persons served by residential setting		
	1991	**1995**	**2002**
Setting by size	2,018 (100%)	1,577 (100%)	3,073 (100%)
16+ Persons	572 (28.3%)	191 (12.1%)	43 (1.4)
7-15 Persons	187 (9.3%)	298 (18.9%)	247 (8.0%)
≤6 Persons	1,259 (62.4%)	1,088 (69%)	2,783 (90.6%)

Source: Prouty, Robert W., Gary Smith and K. Charlie Lakin, *Residential Services for Persons with Developmental Disabilities: Status and Trends Through 2002.* Research and Training Center on Community Living. University of Minnesota, June 2003. [Http://rtc.umn.edu/risp].

[2] Ibid.

TRENDS IN HOME AND COMMUNITY-BASED CARE

As the number and size of larger facilities has decreased over the years, the state has made significant use of Medicaid financing for community-based care. Maine uses one optional service — day habitation; one Section 1915(c) waiver, which includes day habilitation; and some state-funded programs to support community-based care. Day habilitation services are available to persons who meet the ICF/MR eligibility criteria. The service originally was designed to serve people with developmental disabilities who live in nursing homes and need special services due to their conditions.

The state's *Home and Community Based Waiver Services for Persons with Mental Retardation* serves people who would otherwise be in an institution. It provides residential training in a licensed home, including personal support, day habilitation, supported employment, respite, environmental modification, crisis intervention, and other services. About 2,200 people received services in FY2002. Costs are limited to 100% of the aggregate average cost of ICF/MR facilities across the state (approximately $110,000 in 2003).

Chapter 7

FINANCING OF LONG-TERM CARE IN MAINE

In most states, Medicaid is the chief source of financing for long-term care. In Maine, long-term care spending accounted for about 30% of total Medicaid spending in FY2001. In addition, Maine has a number of state-financed programs that complement Medicaid programs. Maine's Medicaid spending on institutional care declined during the 1990s while spending on home and community-based services rose rather dramatically.

MEDICAID SPENDING IN MAINE

Medicaid is a significant part of state budgets. After elementary, secondary and higher education spending, Medicaid spending was the largest share of state budgets in 2001. According to data compiled by the National Association of State Budget Officers (NASBO), *federal and state* Medicaid spending represented almost 20% of state budgets for the United States as a whole in 2001.

In Maine, Medicaid spending is the largest single category of *federal and state* spending. Of the state's $5.3 billion budget in 2001, federal and state Medicaid spending represented one out of every four dollars. Federal and state spending for Medicaid increased from almost 15% of total spending in 1990, and in 2001 at 24.9%, was about equal to spending for elementary, secondary, and higher education combined (**Table 8**).

Table 8. Share of State Spending by Category, Maine and the United States, 1990-2001

Expenditure category	Maine				U.S. total
	1990	1995	2000	2001	2001
Total expenditures (in millions)	$2,651	$3,825	$4,847	$5,269	$1,024,439
Medicaid	14.9%	23.0%	25.0%	24.9%	19.6%
Elementary and secondary education	26.4%	13.9%	19.8%	20.4%	22.2%
Higher education	6.7%	4.4%	4.2%	4.6%	11.3%
Public assistance	6.9%	5.9%	3.4%	2.7%	2.2%
Corrections	2.4%	1.8%	2.0%	1.9%	3.7%
Transportation	10.8%	8.7%	8.6%	8.7%	8.9%
All other expenses	31.9%	42.2%	36.9%	36.8%	32.1%

Source: CRS calculations based on National Association of State Budget Officers (NASBO) State Expenditures Reports 1990-2001.

State Spending for Medicaid services in Maine contributed from state funds *only* (excluding federal funds)[1] increased over 3 times from 1990 to 2001. As a percent of spending for all categories of state spending, state Medicaid spending increased from 6.4% in 1990 to 12% in 2001 (**Table 9**).

Table 9. State spending for Medicaid as a Percent of Total State Spending, Maine and the United States, 1990-2001

State spending	Maine				All states
	1990	1995	2000	2001	2001
Total state spending (in millions)[a]	$2,009	$2,753	$3,352	$3,729	$760,419
State Medicaid spending (millions)[b]	$130	$275	$416	$447	$85,141
State Medicaid spending as a percent of total state spending	6.4%	10.0%	12.4%	12.0%	11.2%

[a] Total state spending for all categories, excluding federal funds.

[b] State spending for Medicaid, exclusive of federal funds.

Source: CRS calculations based on data from the National Association of State Budget Officers (NASBO), State Expenditure Reports for 1991, 1997 and 2001. Data reported are for state fiscal years.

[1] Federal and state governments share the costs of Medicaid spending according to a statutory formula based on a state's relative per capita income (federal medical assistance percentage, or FMAP). In FY2001, the federal share for Medicaid in Maine was 66.12%.

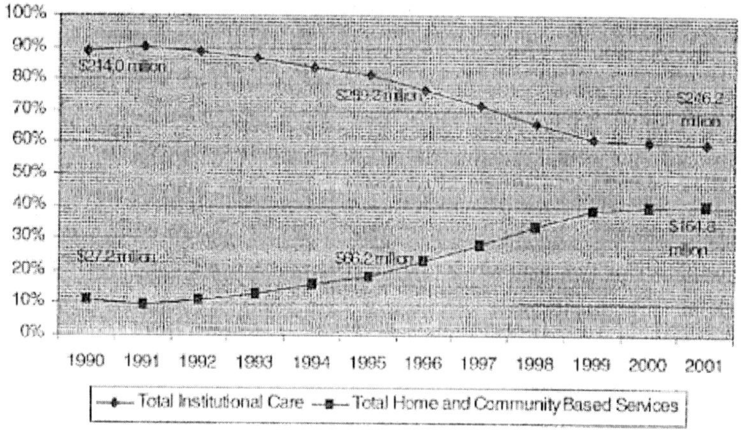

Figure 2. Institutional and Home and Community-Based Services as a Percent of Medicaid Long-Term Care Spending in Maine, 1990-2001.

Source: CRS calculations based on Burwell, *Medicaid Expenditures FY1991-FY2001,* 1990 total Medicaid spending, based on HCFA 64 data provided by the Urban institute, Washington, DC.

Chapter 8

MEDICAID LONG-TERM CARE SPENDING IN MAINE

Long-term care spending represented 30.5% of all Medicaid spending in Maine in FY2001, a significant decrease from 55.1% in 1990 (**Table 10**). This reduction is due to the state's pre-admission screening process for nursing home applicants; restrictions on functional eligibility criteria for Medicaid nursing home coverage; and increased use of home and community-based alternatives to nursing home care that the state started providing in the wake of a mid-1990s state budget crisis. During the same period, spending for home and community-based services as a proportion of total long-term care spending grew almost fourfold to reach 40.1% of long-term care spending in FY2001. Nevertheless, institutional care still dominates long-term care spending and is a significant share of these expenditures at 60%.

In FY2001, $246.2 million or 18.2% of all Medicaid spending was for care in institutions but nursing home spending accounted for 81.8% of total institutional spending (**Table 11**). In the same year, home and community-based services accounted for 12.2% of all Medicaid spending.

Table 10. Medicaid Long-Term Care Spending in Maine, FY1990-FY2001

Maine	FY1990	FY1995	FY2000	FY2001
Long-term spending as a % of Medicaid spending	55.1%	37.5%	32.0%	30.5%
Institutional care spending as % of long-term care spending	88.7%	81.4%	60.2%	59.9%
Nursing home spending as a % of long-term care spending	65.5%	66.7%	51.2%	49.0%
ICFs/MR* spending as a % of long-term care spending	23.2%	14.7%	9.0%	10.9%
Total home and community-based services spending as a % of long-term care spending	11.3%	18.6%	39.8%	40.1%
HCBS waivers spending as a % of long-term care spending	7.8%	14.7%	36.2%	37.2%

*Intermediate care facilities for the mentally retarded.

Source: CRS calculations based on CMS/HCFA 64 data provide by The Medstat Group, Inc. For 2000 and 2001, Burwell Brian et al., *Medicaid Long-Term Care Expenditures in FY2001,* May 10, 20002. For 1995, Brian Burwell, *Medicaid Long-Term Care Expenditures in FY2000,* May 7, 2001. For 1990, Brian Burwell, *Medicaid Expenditures for FY1991.* Systemetrics/McGraw-Hill Healthcare Management Group, Jan.10, 1992, 1990 total Medicaid spending based on HCFA 64 data provided by Urban Institute, Washington, DC. (Hereafter cited as Burwell, *Medicaid Expenditures FY1991-FY2001.*)

Table 11. Medicaid Spending in Maine, Total Spending and Long-Term Care Spending, by Category, FY1990-FY2001 (Dollars in Millions)

Spending category	FY1990 (current dollars)	FY1995 (current dollars)	FY2000 (current dollars)	FY2001 (current dollars)	Percent change FY1990-FY2001 (in constant 2001 dollars)
Total Medicaid	437.8	948.9	1,218.5	1,349.7	142.4%
Total long-term care	241.1	355.5	390.2	411.0	34.1%
Total institutional care	*214.0*	*289.2*	*234.9*	*246.3*	*-9.5%*
Nursing homes	158.0	237.1	199.6	201.4	0.3%
ICFs/MR*	56.0	52.1	35.3	44.8	-37.0%
Total home and community based services	*27.2*	*66.2*	*155.3*	*164.8*	*376.9%*
Home health	5.9	12.2	9.4	6.6	-12.2%
Personal care	2.3	2.0	4.8	5.3	78.9%
HCBS waivers	18.9	52.1	141.1	152.8	535.9%

* Intermediate care facilities for the mentally retarded.

Source: CRS calculations based on Burwell, *Medicaid Expenditures FY1991-FY2001.* Total 1990 Medicaid spending, based on HCFA 64 data provided by the Urban Institute, Washington, DC.

Figures 3 and **4** depict dramatic changes in long-term care spending patterns from FY1990 to FY2001. In FY1990, 23.2% of Medicaid long-term care spending was devoted to care for persons with developmental disabilities in ICFs/MR; this decreased to 10.9% in FY2001. The proportion of Medicaid long-term care spending on nursing home services also declined during that time period from 65.5% to 49.0%. Spending on home and community services increased from 11.3% to 40.1% of long-term care expenditures, primarily due to the expansion of Section 1915(c) waivers, which increased 536% from FY1990 to FY2001 (in constant 2001 dollars).

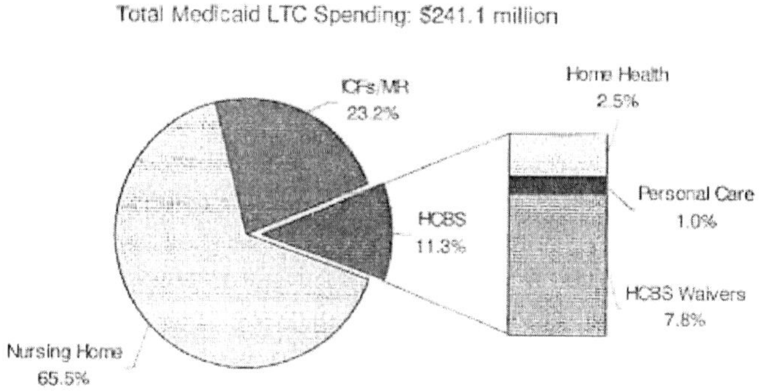

Figure 3. Medicaid Long-Term Care Spending in Maine by Category, FY1990.

Source: CRS calculations based on Burwell, *Medicaid Expenditures FY1991-FY2001.*

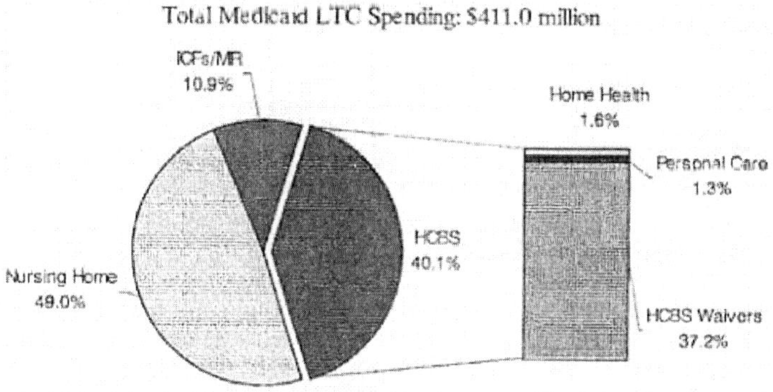

Figure 4. Medicaid Long-Term Care Spending in Maine by Category, FY2001.

Source: CRS calculations based on Burwell, *Medicaid Expenditures FY1991-FY2001.*

Increased funding for Section 1915(c) waiver services does not affect all populations equally. In FY2001, about 15.6% of waiver spending in Maine was devoted to services for the aged and younger persons with disabilities; spending for persons with mental retardation and developmental disabilities accounted for 84.4% of waiver spending in FY2001.

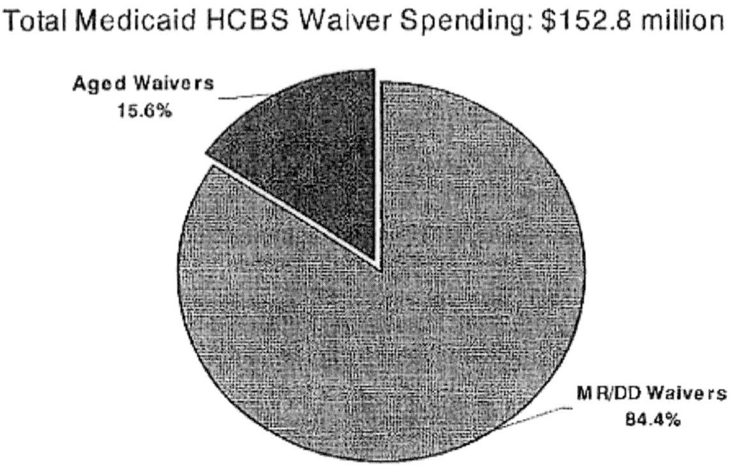

Figure 5. Medicaid Home and Community-Based Services Waiver Spending by Target Population in Maine, FY2001.

Source: CRS calculations based on *Medicaid HCBS Waiver Expenditures, FY1995 through FY2001* by Steve Eiken and Brian Burwell, The Medstat Group, Inc., May 13, 2002.

Medicaid Long-Term Spending in Maine at a Glance

In FY2001, about 30% of Medicaid dollars were spent on long-term care. This as a decline from FY1990 when long-term care represented over 55% of Medicaid spending.

This decline is largely attributed to a decline in spending for nursing home care. This spending represented 15% of total Medicaid spending in FY2001 — a decline from the 36% it represented in FY1990. Nursing home spending grew less than one percent over the period.

As a percent of Medicaid long-term care spending, nursing home care declined from 65.5% to 49% FY1990 to FY2001. During the same period, the portion spent on ICFs/MR decreased from 23.2% to 10.9%.

At the same time, spending on home and community based services increased by almost 400% from FY1990 to FY2001. Home and community-based services represented 40% of long-term care spending in FY2001.

MEDICAID AND STATE SPENDING ON SERVICES FOR PERSONS WITH MENTAL RETARDATION

Federal and state spending for persons with mental retardation and developmental disabilities was $216.8 million in 2000 (**Table 12**). This represented an increase of 812.2% (in constant 2000 dollars) since 1990. Of total 2000 spending, 34.8% was contributed by state resources. Section 1915(c) waiver funding increased from $9.2 million in 1990 to $84.8 million in 2000.

Table 12. Federal and State Spending for Institutional and Community Services for Persons with Mental Retardation/Developmental Disabilities in Maine, 1990 and 2000

	1990 (current dollars)	2000 (current dollars)	Percent of FY2000 total	Percent change (in constant 2000 dollars)
Total funds	79.6	216.8	100%	812.2%
Congregate/institutional services	31.4	9.4	4.4%	-75.8%
Federal funds	17.5	6.3	2.9%	-71.2%
State funds	14.0	3.2	1.5%	-81.6%
Home and community-based services	48.2	207.4	95.6%	246.7%
Federal funds	29.0	135.2	62.3%	275.0%
ICF/MR funds	12.7	16.8	7.8%	7.0%
HCBS waiver	9.2	84.8	39.1%	640.9%
Title XX/SSBG funds	0.9	0.8	0.4%	-29.6%
Other	6.2	32.8	15.1%	323.4%
State funds	19.1	72.2	33.3%	203.8%

Source: CRS calculations based on data presented in *The State of the States in Developmental Disabilities* (Fifth Edition), by David Braddock et al., (1998) Washington, DC, American Association on Mental Retardation, p. 404 (for 1990 data). Unpublished data furnished by Richard Hemp, University of Colorado (for 2000 data).

As discussed earlier, Maine has devoted considerable effort to increasing services in home and community-based settings to persons with developmental disabilities. Table 11 shows that in 2000, 95.6% of total spending was for home and community-based services — $207.4 million. Of total spending in 2000, 39.1% was from waiver programs. This spending increased by 640.9% in constant 2000 dollars since 1990. The state has used waivers to maximize federal Medicaid reimbursement for home and community-based services, while it has dramatically decreased federal spending for institutional services. Federal spending for institutional services decreased by 71.2% in constant dollars from 1990 to 2000.

Chapter 9

ISSUES IN LONG-TERM CARE IN MAINE

The following discussion highlights selected issues raised in state reports collected for this section and in interviews with state officials and key stakeholders conducted during the site visit to Maine in the summer of 2002.

BUDGETARY CONCERNS

In dealing with prior budgetary dilemmas the state has followed a "Medicaid maximization" policy in providing home and community-based care. That is, because the state has opted to take opportunities to provide a number of optional home and community-based services that are allowed under the federal law, it can therefore draw down federal Medicaid matching dollars to support its program.

One of the challenges the state faces during its budgetary crisis is to hold on to the gains it has made in providing home and community services to people with disabilities. According to interviewees, this is particularly the case when the state's nursing home lobby competes with other groups for funding. Part of the state government's plan to close its budget gap would involve a 6% "nursing home bed tax," which would raise $7 million.[1] The money would be used to draw down federal Medicaid funds, which would then go to wages for long-term care workers, including providers other than nursing homes.

---

[1] Rankin Joe, "Governor Proposes Nursing Home Tax," *Kennebec Journal*, June 29, 2002.

Other budget actions would shift some state funded residential costs to Medicaid and reduce spending on state-funded services, including homemaker, adult day services, and Alzheimer's respite care. The Governor's budget proposal would decrease nursing facilities' cost of living adjustment from 3% to 2%.[2] According to state officials, as of March 2002, home and community-based services had not been affected too negatively by budget cuts.

LABOR ISSUES

The health labor shortage is a critical problem affecting all areas of health care, including long-term care and care for persons with developmental disabilities, particularly in Southern Maine. The labor shortage also makes it difficult to recruit state and privately-employed case managers.

Interviewees cited several reasons for the labor shortage. Fourteen percent of Maine's population is aged 65 or over and many younger people are leaving the state to find employment. Interviewees also cited low wages and lack of health insurance as barriers to employment in the long-term care sector. The state has considered becoming a self-insurer for agencies contracting with the state to provide an opportunity for them to participate in a large group health insurance plan.

The results of the labor shortage include high staff turnover and reliance on temporary agency staff. This can disrupt continuity of care in facilities and lead to staff having insufficient training to handle some of the complex needs of nursing home residents. There is also a shortage of experienced nursing home administrators so many come to their jobs with very little training. State officials said that some people in southern Maine may have to be placed on waiting lists for home and community services because of the labor shortage.

Conducting criminal background checks on long-term care employees is another controversial labor issue in Maine. Not all long-term care programs require criminal background checks for long-term care workers and consumer-directed programs have actively resisted this. The state's certified nurse aide registry does not allow people who have committed crimes in health care settings to be on the registry but criminals with other types of

---

[2] Michael O' D. Moore, "Health Professionals Wary of King Cuts," *Bangor Daily News*, June 27, 2002.

convictions can be. Some officials recommended more attention to registries of nurse aides. State officials noted that a U.S.-wide registry could prevent criminals working in long-term care from going from state to state when they lose their credentials.

Consumer Direction

A number of controversial issues raised during the site visit related to various aspects of the consumer-directed programs. Control of these programs was transferred from the Maine Department of Human Services (DHS) to the Department of Labor (DoL) in 2001. The transfer occurred as a result of advocacy efforts on the part of consumers. Many believed that Maine DoL would be the more appropriate administering agency since it has experience with rehabilitation services and independent living services for persons with severe disabilities, (DoL administers programs authorized under the Rehabilitation Act of 1973, including vocational rehabilitation and centers for independent living programs).

Another controversy surrounds paying family members to work for beneficiaries. According to interviewees, this can become problematic when the family members come to consider the payments part of their rights and income, and when families provide inadequate or substandard services. There is also the feeling among some that women who receive payment will become the next generation of poor women because they do not have access to employment that provides fringe benefits (like retirement and health insurance).

Assisted Living Facilities

Some stakeholders interviewed said that assisted living facilities (ALFs) are becoming more popular than nursing homes. However, sometimes people enter nursing homes because federal money isn't available for assisted living facilities. Also, assisted living facilities are supposed to provide personal care as part of the payment they receive from Medicaid but some do not. The ALF regulations give residents the right to age in place but providers say that this is not reflected in the level of Medicaid reimbursement they receive.

WAITING LIST

As of the summer of 2002, the waiting list for residential care for persons with developmental disabilities was 500. People who are in crisis situations move off of the list to receive services first. The waiting list for supported employment was between 300 and 400.

Appendix 1

MAJOR HOME AND COMMUNITY-BASED LONG-TERM CARE PROGRAMS FOR THE ELDERLY AND PERSONS WITH DISABILITIES IN MAINE

Major Home and Community-Based Long-Term Care Programs for the Elderly and Persons with Disabilities in Maine

Program	Target group	Functional eligibility		Financial eligibility		Services	No, of persons enrolled/slots approved and expenditures (SFY2001)	Annual cost cap (aggregate/ individual)	Administrative oversight	Financial oversight
		Criteria	Determined by	Income/ resource limits	Determined by					
Home health (adults only) (Medicaid state plan service)	Adults age 18+	Need for skilled nursing or therapy, homebound, and physician ordered	Home health agency does assessment	100% of poverty; assets of $2,000 or less with additional exclusions in certain circumstances	Bureau of Family Independence	Nursing, therapies, home health aide, psychiatric monitoring	2,238 persons $5,329,567	None	Bureau of Elder and Adult Services	Department of Human Services
Private duty nursing (adults only) (Medicaid state plan service)	Adults age 18+	Limited assistance and one person physical support in two of seven ADLs or cueing in four ADLs	Assessing Services Agency	100% of poverty; assets of $2,000 or less with additional exclusions in certain circumstances	Bureau of Family Independence	Nursing, home health aide, and personal care assistance	1,188 persons $4,292,745	$3,884 a month or, if ventilator dependent, $20,100 a month	Bureau of Elder and Adult Services	Department of Human Services
Personal care services (adults only) (Medicaid state plan service)	Adults age 18 and over	Limited assistance and one person physical support in two of seven ADLS or cueing in four ADLs	Assessing Services Agency	100% of poverty; assets of $2,000 or less with additional exclusions in certain circumstances	Bureau of Family Independence	Nursing, home health aide, and personal care assistance	1,388 persons $4,986,955	$3,884 a month or, if ventilator dependent, $20,100 a month	Bureau of Elder and Adult Services	Department of Human Services

Major Home and Community-Based Long-Term Care Programs for the Elderly and Persons with Disabilities in Maine (Continued)

Program	Target group	Functional eligibility		Financial eligibility		Services	No, of persons enrolled/slots approved and expenditures (SFY2001)	Annual cost cap (aggregate/ individual)	Administrative oversight	Financial oversight
		Criteria	Determined by	Income/ resource limits	Determined by					
Adult day health services (Medicaid state plan service)	18 and older	Limited assistance and one person physical support in two of seven ADLs or cueing in four ADLs	Day care provider or Assessing Services Agency	100% of poverty; assets of $2,000 or less with additional exclusions in certain circumstances	Bureau of Family Independence	Monitoring of health care, nursing rehabilitation counseling, exercise, health promotion	173 persons $787,015	Must attend a minimum of 4 hours weekly	Bureau of Elder and Adult services	Department of Human Services
Consumer-directed personal care (Medicaid state plan service)	18 and older	Limited assistance and one person physical support in two ADLs and cognitively capable of self direction	Alpha One or Assessing Services Agency	100% of poverty; assets of $2,000 or less with additional exclusions in certain circumstances	Bureau of Family Independence	Personal care assistance, skills training	357 persons $4.1 million	Up to 35 hours a week plus less than 14 night-time hours a week	Alpha One	Department of Labor

Major Home and Community-Based Long-Term Care Programs for the Elderly and Persons with Disabilities in Maine (Continued)

Program	Target group	Functional eligibility		Financial eligibility		Services	No, of persons enrolled/slots approved and expenditures (SFY2001)	Annual cost cap (aggregate/ individual)	Administrative oversight	Financial oversight
		Criteria	Determined by	Income/ resource limits	Determined by					
Consumer-directed waiver (Medicaid 1915(c) waiver)	18 and older	Nursing facility eligible and cognitively capable of self direction	Alpha One or Assessing Services Agency	222% of poverty; and assets of $2,000 or less with additional exclusions in certain circumstances	Bureau of Family Independence	Case management with skills training and consumer directed personal care assistants	279 persons $8.3 million	90% of average nursing facility payment	Alpha One	Department of Labor

Major Home and Community-Based Long-Term Care Programs for the Elderly and Persons with Disabilities in Maine (Continued)

Program	Target group	Functional eligibility		Financial eligibility		Services	No, of persons enrolled/slots approved and expenditures (SFY2001)	Annual cost cap (aggregate/ individual)	Administrative oversight	Financial oversight
		Criteria	Determined by	Income/ resource limits	Determined by					
Elder and waiver (Medicaid 1915(c) waiver	Age 18 and older	Nursing facility eligible	Assessing Services Agency	222% of poverty and assets of $2,000 or less with additional exclusions in certain circumstances	Bureau of Family Independence	Case management, nursing home health aide, certified nursing assistants, therapies, personal care assistant, homemaker, adult day health care, emergency response systems, mental health, transportation respite	1,589 persons $19,096,433	100% of average nursing facility payment	Bureau of Elder and Adult Services	Department of Human Services

Major Home and Community-Based Long-Term Care Programs for the Elderly and Persons with Disabilities in Maine (Continued)

Program	Target group	Functional eligibility		Financial eligibility		Services	No, of persons enrolled/slots approved and expenditures (SFY2001)	Annual cost cap (aggregate/ individual)	Administrative oversight	Financial oversight
		Criteria	Determined by	Income/ resource limits	Determined by					
Residential care: medical and remedial component (Medicaid and state funded)	Age 18 and older	Needs shelter and support	Residential care provider	Income limit varies with facility rate; assets of $2,000 or less	Bureau of Family Independence	Room and board, medical and remedial services	4,325 $45.1 million	Personal needs allowance of up to $70 a month	Bureau of Elder and Adult Services	Department of Human Services
Residential care: room and board (Medicaid and state funded)	Age 18 and older	Needs shelter and support	Residential care provider	Income limit varies with facility rate; assets of $2,000 or less	Bureau of Family Independence	Room and board, medical and remedial services	4,403 $16,698,724	Personal needs allowance of up to $70 a month	Bureau of Elder and Adult Services	Department of Human Services
Congregate housing program (state funded)	18 and older	three IADLs, two ADLs, or one ADL and two IADLs	Provider	$50,000 asset limit	Bureau of Family Independence	Service coordination, chore services, one meal a day	260 $592,156	Based on needs of resident	Bureau of Elder and Adult Services	Department of Human Services

Major Home and Community-Based Long-Term Care Programs for the Elderly and Persons with Disabilities in Maine (Continued)

Program	Target group	Functional eligibility: Criteria	Functional eligibility: Determined by	Financial eligibility: Income/ resource limits	Financial eligibility: Determined by	Services	No, of persons enrolled/slots approved and expenditures (SFY2001)	Annual cost cap (aggregate/ individual)	Administrative oversight	Financial oversight
Assisted living CHSP (state funded)	18 and older	three IADLs, two ADLs, or one ADL and two IADLs	Provider	$50,000 asset limit	Bureau of Family Independence	Service coordination, chore services, one meal a day	199 $1,812,206	Based on needs of resident	Bureau of Elder and Adult Services	Department of Human Services
Adult foster homes (state funded)	18 and older	Needs shelter and support	Provider	$14 gross income and assets of $2,000 or less	Bureau of Family Independence	Medicaid and remedial services, room and board	Not available	Resident pays maximum of $544 a month. Personal needs allowance of up to $70 a month	Bureau of Elder and Adult Services	Department of Human Services
Adult family care homes (Medicaid and state funded)	18 and older	Cueing in four ADLs; cognitive or behavioral problems with two or four ADLs	Provider	$1,706 gross income and assets of $2,000 or less	Bureau of Family Independence	Medicaid and remedial services, room and board	Not available	Based on needs of resident. Personal needs allowance of up to $70 a month	Bureau of Elder and Adult Services	Department of Human Services

Major Home and Community-Based Long-Term Care Programs for the Elderly and Persons with Disabilities in Maine (Continued)

Program	Target group	Functional eligibility		Financial eligibility		Services	No, of persons enrolled/slots approved and expenditures (SFY2001)	Annual cost cap (aggregate/ individual)	Administrative oversight	Financial oversight
		Criteria	Determined by	Income/ resource limits	Determined by					
Home-based care (state funded)	18 and older	Total of three limitations with at least one ADL or cueing in four ADLs	Assessing Services Agency	No upper limit. Copayment of 4% of monthly income and 3% of assets exceeding $15,000	Bureau of Family Independence	Case management, nursing home health aide, certified nursing assistants, therapies, personal care assistant, homemaker, adult day health care, emergency response systems, mental health, transportation respite	3,863 persons $12,4 million	85% of nursing facility rate ($3,301 in SFY2002)	Elder Independence of Maine	Department of Human Services

Major Home and Community-Based Long-Term Care Programs for the Elderly and Persons with Disabilities in Maine (Continued)

Program	Target group	Functional eligibility		Financial eligibility		Services	No, of persons enrolled/slots approved and expenditures (SFY2001)	Annual cost cap (aggregate/ individual)	Administrative oversight	Financial oversight
		Criteria	Determined by	Income/ resource limits	Determined by					
Home-based care: consumer-directed (state funded)	18 and older	Total of three limitations with at least one ADL and cognitively capable of self direction	Assessing Services Agency or Alpha One	No upper limit. Copayment of 4% of monthly income and 3% of assets exceeding $30,000	Bureau of Family Independence	Personal care assistance and skills training	203 $3,118,374	100% of nursing facility rate ($3,884 a month in SFY2002)	Alpha One	Department of Labor
Adult day services (state funded)	18 and older	One ADL or cueing with four ADLs	Day care provider or assessing services agency	$50,000 asset test. Copayment of 20% of cost of services		Monitor health care, nursing rehabilitation counseling, exercise, health promotion	119 $304,240	Attend a minimum of 4 hours a week	Alpha One	Department of Labor

Major Home and Community-Based Long-Term Care Programs for the Elderly and Persons with Disabilities in Maine (Continued)

Program	Target group	Functional eligibility		Financial eligibility		Services	No, of persons enrolled/slots approved and expenditures (SFY2001)	Annual cost cap (aggregate/ individual)	Administrative oversight	Financial oversight
		Criteria	Determined by	Income/ resource limits	Determined by					
Alzheimer's respite (state and Older Americans Act funded)	18 and older	Need-based	Bureau of Elder and Adult Services/Area Agencies in Aging	$50,000 asset test. Copayment of 20% of cost of services		In-home or institutional respite, adult day care respite	430 $754,609	$3,800 a year	Bureau of Elder and Adult Services	Department of Human Services
Homemaker (state funded)	21 and older	Need help with three IADLs and one ADL	Homemaker provider or assessing services agency	$50,000 asset test. Copayment of 20% of services		Homemaking, chore, grocery shopping, laundry, incidental personal care, transportation	1,664 $2,553,199	Ten hours a month	Home Resources of Maine or Aroostook Home Health Services	Department of Human Services

Major Home and Community-Based Long-Term Care Programs for the Elderly and Persons with Disabilities in Maine (Continued)

Program	Target group	Functional eligibility		Financial eligibility		Services	No, of persons enrolled/slots approved and expenditures (SFY2001)	Annual cost cap (aggregate/ individual)	Administrative oversight	Financial oversight
		Criteria	Determined by	Income/ resource limits	Determined by					
Home and community based waiver services for persons with mental retardation (Medicaid 1915(c) waiver)	All ages	ICF/MR level of care	Department of Behavioral and Developmental Services, Adult Mental Retardation Services	300% of the SSI level; $2,000 per individual	Department of Human Services, Bureau of Family Independence	Residential training services in a DHS licensed home Personal support services Day habilitation services Supported employment Respite care Environmental modification, communication assessment Crisis intervention Consultative services	2,200 slots	100% of the average aggregate costs of ICF/MR facilities (approx. $110,000 per year in 2003)	Department of Behavioral and Developmental Services, Adult Mental Retardation Services	Department of Human Services

Appendix 2

POPULATION IN LARGE STATE FACILITIES

Table A-2. Population in Large State Facilities for Persons with Mental Retardation/Developmental Disabilities and Closure Date, Maine

Large state MR/DD facilities or units operating 1908-1998	Year facility opened	Year closed
Aroostook Residential Center (Presque Isle)	1972	
Elizabeth Levinson Center (Bangor)	1971	
Freeport Town Square	not available	
Pineland Center (Pownal)	1908	1995

Source: Residential Services for Persons with Developmental Disabilities: Status and Trends Through 2001, Research and Training Center on Community Living, Institute on Community Integration/UCEED, University of Minnesota, June 2002; and personal communication with personnel of the Department of Behavioral and Developmental Services.

Appendix 3

About the Census Population Projections

The projections use the cohort-component method. The cohort-component method requires separate assumptions for each component of population change: births, deaths, internal migration (internal migration refers to state-to-state migration, domestic migration, or interstate migration), and international migration... . The projection's starting date is July 1, 1994. The national population total is consistent with the middle series of the Census Bureau's national population projections for the years 1996 to 2025. *Source:* Paul R. Campbell, 1996, *Population Projections for States by Age, Sex, Race, and Hispanic Origin: 1995 to 2025,* U.S. Bureau of the Census, Population Division, PPL-47. For detailed explanation of the methodology, see same at [http://www.census.gov/population/www/projections/ppl47.html].

ACKNOWLEDGMENTS

The editor wishes to acknowledge the generous time and contributions of the many state officials and stakeholders who provided information on long-term care services in Maine. Without their generous time and invaluable experience and insight, this book would not be possible. We would particularly like to thank officials from the Department of Human Services, the Department of Behavioral and Developmental Services, and the Department of Labor. We would also like to thank the advocates and providers who offered valuable perspectives on the long-term care system in Maine.

The editor also gratefully acknowledge the excellent assistance of Flora Adams and Charlotte Foote in the productions of this section.

INDEX

H

I

K

L

M

N

O

P

R

S

T

W